THE THYROID COOKBOOK

Thyroid-Friendly Meals for Improved Energy and Wellness

Antone Blick

COPYRIGHT

TABLE OF CONTENTS

INTRODUCTION 7

RECIPES 9

Oven Baked Pumpkin Spice Pancakes 9

Apple Pork Medallions 10

Slow Cooker Chicken and Squash Soup 12

Roasted Grape Chicken Thighs 13

Banana and Cream "Oatmeal" 14

Coconut Blueberry Paleo Oatmeal 15

Butternut Squash and Apple Hash with Sausage 16

Aip tigernut granola 18

Poached Tilapia 19

Golden Milk Quinoa Porridge 20

Paleo Chicken Curry Soup 22

Vegetable frittata 24

Gluten-free chicken and vegetable pie 25

Chicken Ratatouille 27

Eggplant, Chickpea, and Chard Shakshuka 29

Beef and pearl barley salad with fresh chimichurri 31

Banana-Hazelnut Smoothie 32

Cauliflower and celeriac soup...33

Chai-spiced Smoothie Bowl 34

Cinnamon oat & almond loaf..35

Chicken & herb meatball soup..37

Chicken and parsley salad pitas 38

Barbecued chilli mint lamb and tomato salad 40

Chickpea curry with pumpkin and baby spinach...............................42

Berry sundae 43

Vegetable frittata..44

Gluten-free chicken and vegetable pie 45

Sautéed Shrimp 47

Spaghetti squash with chunky tomato sauce 48

Savory Pumpkin Hummus 50

Mediterranean Deviled Eggs 51

Maple and Apple Pork Chops...52

Basil chicken bites...53

Spanish Paella with Shrimp and Scallops..54

Stuffed pork tenderloin with collard greens 55

Grilled Salmon Fillet with Chili-Infused Blackberry Sauce..............57

Sesame-Ginger Grilled Salmon 58

Grilled Romaine and Asparagus Salad 60

Pineapple Ginger Glazed Baked Salmon 61

Vegetable and Sausage Skillet 62

Layered chicken, lemon and risoni bake 63

Masala egg curry 65

Salsa verde chicken with ricotta-stuffed capsicum 67

Cottage cheese and salad sandwich 68

Crisp-skinned salmon 69

Apple bircher muesli 70

Asian-style Pearl Couscous with grilled salmon 72

Curried Pearl Couscous with pomegranates 73

Fresh kale, avocado and pomegranate salad 75

Asparagus, corn and brazil nut salad 76

Avocado & Cottage Cheese Whip on Toast 77

Turmeric Ginger Ground Turkey Bowls 78

Paleo Banana Bread 80

Salmon With Cilantro-Lime Salsa 82

Salmon Seaweed Wraps 84

Roasted Dijon Lamb With Herbs and Country Vegetables 86

Fajita-Seasoned Grilled Chicken 87

Grilled Salmon Salad 88

Spiced Citrus Tea 89

Avocado Salsa..90

Balsamic Grilled Pork Chops..91

Lemon Pepper Chicken Wings 92

Rainbow Roots Slaw with Tahini Parsley Dressing 93

Broccoli Italian Style 94

Orange-Pomegranate Glazed Ham 95

Banana Blueberry Muffins – Nut Free 96

INTRODUCTION

The thyroid gland is a small organ that's located in the front of the neck, wrapped around the windpipe (trachea). It's shaped like a butterfly, smaller in the middle with two wide wings that extend around the side of your throat. The thyroid is a gland. You have glands throughout your body, where they create and release substances that help your body do a specific thing. Your thyroid makes hormones that help control many vital functions of your body.

When your thyroid doesn't work properly, it can impact your entire body. If your body makes too much thyroid hormone, you can develop a condition called hyperthyroidism. If your body makes too little thyroid hormone, it's called hypothyroidism. Both conditions are serious and need to be treated by your healthcare provider.

Your thyroid has an important job to do within your body — releasing and controlling thyroid hormones that control metabolism. Metabolism is a process where the food you take into your body is transformed into energy. This energy is used throughout your entire body to keep many of your body's systems working correctly. Think of your metabolism as a generator. It takes in raw energy and uses it to power something bigger.

The thyroid controls your metabolism with a few specific hormones — T4 (thyroxine, contains four iodide atoms) and T3 (triiodothyronine, contains three iodide atoms). These two hormones are created by the thyroid and they tell the body's cells how much energy to use. When your thyroid works properly, it will maintain the right amount of hormones to keep your metabolism working at the right rate. As the hormones are used, the thyroid creates replacements.

RECIPES

Oven Baked Pumpkin Spice Pancakes

Ingredients

☐ 2 tablespoons gelatin

☐ ½ cup hot water

☐ 4 medjool dates, pits removed

☐ ½ cup pumpkin puree

☐ 2 tablespoons melted coconut oil

☐ 1 teaspoon apple cider vinegar

☐ ⅔ cup sweet potato flour

☐ 1 teaspoon baking soda

☐ ½ teaspoon salt

☐ 1 teaspoon cinnamon

Directions

1. Preheat oven to 350°F and line a cookie sheet with parchment paper or a silicone mat.

2. Dissolve the gelatin in the hot water and mix well.

3. In a food processor or high speed blender, puree dates, pumpkin, coconut oil, apple cider vinegar, and the gelatin and water mixture until smooth.

4. Add sweet potato flour, baking soda, salt and cinnamon. Puree again until all ingredients are well combined (the batter will be thick – more like a cake than a traditional pancake).

Apple Pork Medallions

INGREDIENTS

☐ 2-3 cups peeled and sliced Fuji apples (sliced to ¼" thick)

☐ 1 teaspoon cinnamon

☐ ½ teaspoon + 1 teaspoon salt

☐ 2 tablespoons honey

☐ 2 tablespoons apple cider vinegar

☐ ¼ cup arrowroot starch/flour

☐ 1 teaspoon onion powder

☐ ½ teaspoon garlic powder

☐ 2 tablespoons extra virgin olive oil

☐ 1 lb pork loin/tenderloin, cut into ½" medallions

☐ 2 teaspoon fresh thyme leaves

Directions

1. In a large bowl, mix together apples, cinnamon, ½ teaspoon salt, honey and vinegar. Set aside.

2. In a smaller bowl, mix together arrowroot starch/flour, 1 teaspoon salt, onion powder, and garlic powder.

3. Place olive oil in a large skillet or chef's pan over medium high heat. When oil is heated, dredge the pork medallions in the flour mixture, shaking off excess, then adding to the pan. Brown the medallions on each side, turning only once.

4. Turn heat down to medium low. Add apple mixture and thyme leaves to the pan. Cover, and simmer for 20 minutes. Check once in a while to make sure it doesn't burn. (Depending on your stove, you may need a lower heat.) Serve with a leafy green vegetable and/or something starchy.

Slow Cooker Chicken and Squash Soup

INGREDIENTS

☐ 1 lb raw chicken thighs

☐ 4 cups peeled, chopped butternut squash

☐ 1 cup peeled, chopped carrot

☐ 1 medium yellow onion, chopped

☐ 2 cups chopped mushrooms

☐ 1 teaspoon garlic powder

☐ 1 teaspoon sea salt

☐ 2 tablespoons minced fresh sage

☐ 4 cups chicken bone broth

☐ 2 cups chopped, packed kale (stems removed)

☐ 2 tablespoons lemon juice

Directions

1. Combine all ingredients, except kale and lemon juice, in slow cooker, stir to combine.

2. Cover and cook on high for 4 hours or on low for 7 hours.

3. When coaoking has finished, remove chicken thighs with a slotted spoon. Rough chop chicken (which should easily fall apart).

4. Add chopped chicken, kale, and lemon juice to slow cooker. Stir to combine and wilt kale. Enjoy!

Roasted Grape Chicken Thighs

INGREDIENTS

- ⅓ cup balsamic vinegar

- ⅓ cup + 2 tablespoons extra virgin olive oil, divided

- ½ teaspoon sea salt

- 3 cloves garlic, minced

- 1 tablespoon lemon juice

- 2 teaspoon chopped fresh rosemary

- 4 boneless, skinless chicken thighs

- 2 cups halved seedless grapes

- ½ cup chopped onions

Directions

1. In a medium-sized bowl, whisk together vinegar, ⅓ cup olive oil, salt, garlic, lemon juice, and rosemary. Add

the chicken to the marinade, and turn to coat. Marinate at room temperature for 20 minutes.

2. Preheat oven to 425 degrees F. In an iron skillet or other oven-safe skillet over medium high heat, place 2 tablespoons olive oil. When oil is hot, remove only the chicken thighs to the skillet (reserving marinade), and cook them for 2 minutes on each side.

3. Toss grapes and onions in the reserved marinade, then empty the whole thing into the skillet with the chicken. Carefully place the uncovered skillet in the oven, and bake for 20 minutes.

Banana and Cream "Oatmeal"

Ingredients

☐ 1 ripe banana

☐ 2 tbsp coconut butter

☐ 1 sea salt, just a pinch

☐ ¼ tsp ground cinnamon power

Directions

1. Mash your banana and add the Celtic sea salt and cinnamon.

2. Warm the coconut manna/butter in sauce pan over low heat.

3. When it's runny and warm remove from the heat and scoop it into the banana mixture.

4. Top with your favorite toppings and enjoy!

Coconut Blueberry Paleo Oatmeal

Ingredients

☐ 1 cup full fat organic coconut milk

☐ 2 ripe bananas, broken into pieces medium-large size

☐ ¼ cup coconut butter or coconut manna

☐ 1 pinch sea salt

☐ 1 tbsp grass-fed gelatin

☐ 1 cup fresh blueberries

☐ 1 ¼ - 1 ½ cups finely shredded coconut depends how thick you like your oatmeal

Directions

1. Place a medium pot on the stove on medium heat

2. Add the coconut milk, bananas, coconut butter, and sea salt to the pot

3. Bring to a boil

4. Turn down the heat and simmer for 10 minutes, stirring every couple minutes to break up the banana pieces

5. Add the gelatin and stir well to dissolve

6. Add the blueberries and cook for another 2-3 minutes

7. Remove from heat and add the shredded coconut until it reaches your desired thickness

8. Let sit for approximately 5 minutes to allow the coconut to soften

9. Serve and enjoy!

Butternut Squash and Apple Hash with Sausage

Ingredients

☐ 1½ Tbsp. Coconut oil, divided (or cooking fat of choice – avocado oil or ghee)

☐ 1 medium onion, diced

☐ 1 small butternut squash (1½ lbs.), peeled and cut into ¼-inch dice (about 3 cups)

☐ 1 medium apple, cored and diced

☐ 12 ounces ground turkey or chicken or pork

☐ ½ tsp. Dried sage

☐ ¼ tsp. Dried thyme

☐ ¼ tsp. Garlic powder

☐ ½ tsp. Sea salt (more to taste)

☐ Pinch of nutmeg

☐ Red pepper flakes

☐ 3 cups kale, chard or spinach, washed and torn

Directions

1. Combine ground turkey, sage, thyme, garlic powder, salt and nutmeg or red pepper flakes (if using) in small bowl. Stir with large spoon or use your hands to combine. Set aside.

2. Place a large skillet over medium-high heat. Add 1 tsp. Coconut oil and heat just until oil starts to shimmer. Add onion and butternut squash. Sauté for 7-8 minutes, stirring occasionally.

3. Add 3 Tbsp. Water and diced apple. Cook an additional 5 minutes, stirring occasionally.

4. Move vegetable mixture to one side of the pan. Add remaining coconut oil and turkey mixture. Allow turkey to cook a few minutes before breaking it up with a spatula or wooden spoon.

5. Continue to cook 5-6 minutes or until turkey is cooked through and no longer pink. Stir to combine vegetables and sausage.

6. Place kale/chard/spinach on top of hash and cover with a lid. Allow greens to wilt, about 1-2 minutes. Stir, season with additional salt and pepper and serve.

Aip tigernut granola

INGREDIENTS

☐ 6 oz (165g) tigernuts

☐ 1 oz (30 g) coconut flakes

☐ 2 oz (60 g) mixed dried fruit

☐ 1 Tablespoon (15 ml) honey

Directions

1. Preheat the oven to 350°F / 180°C.

2. Combine the tigernuts, coconut flakes, dried fruit, and honey together in a bowl. Mix until well coated. Spread

out in an even layer on a large roasting tray and place in the oven for 6-7 minutes. Remove the tray from the oven set aside to cool completely.

3. Store in a sealed container.

Poached Tilapia

INGREDIENTS

☐ 5 cups bone broth

☐ ½ teaspoon dried thyme

☐ 1 dried bay leaf

☐ 4 fillets tilapia, about 2 lbs

☐ Salt, to taste

☐ Lemons, to serve

Directions

1. Add the broth and thyme to a frying pan then bring to a boil over high heat.

2. Add 2 fillets to the pan and then let cook 5-6 minutes or until flakey. You may need to flip the tilapia if they are thicker than the broth is deep.

3. Once the first two fillets are finished cooking, carefully transfer them to a platter or serving dish.

4. Next add the remaining two fillets to the pan and let cook for another 5-6 minutes or until flakey.

5. Remove the fillets and carefully add them to the serving dish.

6. At this point the broth should be somewhat cooked down but continue to let boil for another 5 minutes until it's reduced even more.

7. Add salt and lemon, to taste, then pour the sauce over the fillets. Serve immediately.

Golden Milk Quinoa Porridge

INGREDIENTS

☐ 2 cups organic white quinoa rinsed

☐ 2 cups unsweetened coconut milk

☐ 1 teaspoon pure vanilla extract

☐ 1 teaspoon ground turmeric

☐ 1 teaspoon ground cinnamon

☐ ½ teaspoon ground ginger

☐ 1/8 teaspoon black pepper

☐ 1/8 teaspoon salt

☐ ½ cup canned pears with juice, diced

☐ ½ cup golden raisins

☐ ¼ cup unsweetened coconut flakes

Directions

IN THE INSTANT POT

1. In the Instant Pot, combine the washed quinoa and coconut milk. Whisk together well.

2. Set to high pressure and cook for 1 minute. Allow to stand for 10 minutes on natural pressure relief.

3. Carefully remove the lid and stir in the vanilla, turmeric, cinnamon, ginger, black pepper, and salt.

4. Top with pears, raisins, and coconut flakes as desired.

ON THE STOVE TOP

1. Rinse the quinoa under cold water.

2. Combine the quinoa and coconut milk in a medium sauce pan and place over medium heat.

3. Bring to a boil, then reduce the heat to simmer and cover with a tight fitting lid. Cook 10-15 minutes until most of the liquid is absorbed.

4. Remove from the heat and stir in the rest of the ingredients: vanilla, turmeric, cinnamon, ginger, black pepper, and salt.

5. Top with pears, raisins, and coconut flakes as desired.

Paleo Chicken Curry Soup

INGREDIENTS

☐ 1 tablespoon coconut oil

☐ 1 pound organic ground chicken

☐ 2 tablespoons sliced fresh ginger approx. 2″ piece, peeled and thinly sliced

☐ 1 cup diced celery

☐ ½ teaspoon salt

☐ 2 cloves sliced fresh garlic peeled and thinly sliced

☐ 1 cup sliced green onion whites and greens divided

☐ 3 cups stock or broth

☐ ½ cup shredded carrots

☐ 1 teaspoon ground turmeric

☐ 1/16 teaspoon ground cinnamon

☐ ¼ cup packed fresh cilantro

☐ 14.5 ounce can lite coconut milk

☐ ¼ teaspoon crushed red pepper optional

Directions

1. In a large soup pot, heat the coconut oil over medium-high heat.

2. When the oil is hot, add the ground chicken and ginger and cook for 5-10 minutes, or until the chicken begins to brown.

3. Add the celery and ½ teaspoon salt and cook for 2-3 minutes, or until turning translucent.

4. Add the garlic, cook for 1-2 minutes.

5. Add ½ cup white part of green onions, cook 1 minute.

6. Add the mushroom stock, carrots, turmeric, and cinnamon. Turn up the heat and bring to a boil.

7. Once boiling, reduce the heat to simmer, cover with a tight-fitting lid and let cook 20 minutes, stirring occasionally.

8. After 20 minutes, add the ½ cup green part of green onions, cilantro, and coconut milk and turn the heat to high and return to a boil.

9. Let simmer for another 10 minutes before serving.

10. Top with additional fresh cilantro and green onions as desired.

Vegetable frittata

INGREDIENTS

• Olive oil spray

• 1 tablespoon olive oil

• 500g frozen stir-fry vegetable mix, thawed

• 6 eggs

• 125ml (1/2 cup) milk

• Mixed salad leaves, to serve

Directions

1. Preheat oven to 180°C. Spray a 20cm (base measurement) square cake pan with oil. Line base and sides with non-stick baking paper, allowing the 2 long sides to overhang.

2. Heat oil in a large non-stick frying pan over medium-high heat. Stir-fry the vegetables for 3 minutes or until soft. Transfer to the prepared pan.

3. Use a balloon whisk to whisk eggs and milk in a bowl until combined. Season with salt and pepper. Pour over

the vegetables. Bake for 25-30 minutes or until set and light golden.

4. Set aside for 10 minutes to cool slightly. Serve with salad leaves.

Gluten-free chicken and vegetable pie

INGREDIENTS

☐ 1 tablespoon sunflower oil

☐ 1 garlic clove, finely chopped

☐ 400g chicken breast fillets, diced

☐ 1 medium zucchini, chopped

☐ 1 medium carrot, peeled, chopped

☐ 1 medium potato, peeled, diced

☐ 2 cups Massel chicken style liquid stock

☐ 2 tablespoons gluten-free cornflour

☐ ¼ cup chopped fresh flat-leaf parsley leaves

☐ ¼ cup fresh tarragon leaves, finely chopped

GLUTEN-FREE PIE PASTRY

☐ ½ cup rice flour

☐ ½ cup gluten-free cornflour

☐ ¼ cup buckwheat flour

☐ ¼ teaspoon salt

☐ 50g Nuttelex dairy-free spread, chopped

☐ ¼ cup sunflower oil

☐ 1 egg, lightly beaten

Directions

1. Preheat oven to 200C/180C fan-forced. Heat oil in a saucepan over medium heat. Add garlic and chicken. Cook, stirring, for 5 minutes or until browned. Add zucchini, carrot and potato. Cook for 3 minutes. Add 1 cup stock to pan.

2. Place cornflour and ¼ cup remaining stock in a bowl. Stir to form a paste. Stir in remaining stock. Stir cornflour mixture into chicken mixture. Bring to the boil. Reduce heat to medium-low. Simmer for 5 minutes or until just thickened. Stir through parsley and tarragon. Spoon mixture into a 5 cup-capacity ovenproof dish.

3. Make pastry: Sift rice flour, cornflour, buckwheat flour and salt into a large bowl. Add spread, 1 tablespoon cold water and sunflower oil. Using a flat-bladed knife, stir to form a dough, adding extra cold water if needed. Knead

dough for 3 minutes or until smooth and combined. Shape dough into a disc.

4. Roll pastry out on a lightly floured surface until large enough to cover dish. Place pastry over filling. Pinch edges to seal. Brush with egg. Bake for 35 to 40 minutes or until pastry is golden. Stand for 5 minutes to cool. Serve.

Chicken Ratatouille

INGREDIENTS:

☐ 8 bone-in, skin-on chicken thighs, patted dry

☐ Kosher salt

☐ Freshly ground black pepper

☐ tablespoons Garlic-Infused Oil, made with olive oil, or purchased equivalent

☐ ¾ cup (48 g) chopped scallions, green parts only

☐ Pound (455 g) eggplant, trimmed, peeled and cut into 1-inch (2.5 cm) cubes

☐ Pounds (910 g) beefsteak tomatoes, cut into ½-inch (12 mm) dice

☐ medium zucchini, cut into ½-inch (12 mm) dice

☐ 1 red bell pepper, trimmed, cored and roughly chopped

☐ 1tablespoon tomato paste

☐ 1 tablespoon finely chopped fresh thyme or 1 teaspoon dried

☐ ½ teaspoon FreeFod Garlic Replacer, optional

☐ Fresh basil leaves

☐ Fresh thyme

Directions:

1. Season the chicken on all sides with salt and pepper.

2. Heat a large Dutch oven over medium heat. Add about half the oil and heat to shimmering. Add the chicken, skin side down, and cook, without moving, until golden brown and crispy; flip over and cook the second side, about 8 minutes total. Remove chicken from pan and set aside.

3. Add remaining oil, add scallion greens and sauté on low-medium heat until softened. Stir in the eggplant and sauté until it begins to soften, about 5 minutes, then stir in tomatoes, zucchini, red bell pepper, tomato paste, thyme and FreeFod Garlic Replacer, if using. Cook over medium heat, stirring occasionally, until vegetables are tender and mixture has thickened, about 10 minutes

4. Nestle the chicken down into the ratatouille, skin side up, cover, and adjust heat to a simmer. Continue to cook until chicken reaches an internal temperature of 160°F (71°C), about 10 minutes more. Tear fresh basil and/or thyme and scatter over the top right before serving.

Eggplant, Chickpea, and Chard Shakshuka

Ingredients

☐ 2 tablespoons avocado oil

☐ 1 small yellow onion, finely chopped

☐ 1 red bell pepper, finely chopped

☐ 4 cloves garlic

☐ 2 cups eggplant, peeled and chopped

☐ 1 (28-ounce) can crushed tomatoes

☐ 2 tsp ground cumin

☐ 1/8 tsp cayenne pepper

☐ 1/3 cup mild harissa paste

☐ 4 to 6 eggs

☐ 1 head Swiss chard, chopped

☐ 1 (14-ounce) can chickpeas, drained and rinsed

For Serving:

- ☐ 1/3 cup feta cheese crumbles

- ☐ ¼ cup fresh parsley, chopped

- ☐ 4 slices bread of choice, toasted

Directions

1. Add the avocado oil to a 10 or 12-inch cast iron skillet and heat to medium-high.

2. Add the onion, bell pepper and garlic cook, stirring occasionally, until vegetables soften, about 3 minutes. Stir in the eggplant and sauté until golden-brown, about 5 to 8 minutes. Add the diced tomatoes, cumin, cayenne, chili powder and sea salt and bring to a full boil.

3. Add the chopped chard leaves and chickpeas. Cover, and cook until chard has wilted, about 2 to 3 minutes.

4. Dig 4 to 6 wells into the shakshuka mixture and crack eggs into the wells. Reduce heat to medium-low, cover, and cook until the egg whites have set up, about 10 to 15 minutes.

5. Sprinkle with feta cheese and fresh parsley. Serve with toasted bread.

Beef and pearl barley salad with fresh chimichurri

Ingredients

☐ 100 g Beef topside roast, lean, roasted and sliced

☐ 60 g Pearl barley, uncooked

☐ 1 ½ cup Spinach, shredded

☐ ¼ Medium red onion, finely diced

☐ 100 g Cherry tomatoes, halved

☐ Juice and zest of ¼ lemon

☐ 1 tsp Extra virgin olive oil

☐ 1 tsp White wine vinegar

☐ 1 tsp Chopped flat-leaf parsley, finely chopped

☐ 1 tsp Chopped fresh coriander, finely chopped

☐ 1 Garlic clove, crushed

☐ Pinch red chilli flakes

Directions

1. Bring a small pot of water to the boil, and cook the barley for 25 minutes, or until cooked through. Alternatively, you can place it in a microwave-safe bowl,

cover with water, and then place cling film tightly over the bowl. Make a cut in the cling film to allow steam to escape, then microwave on a low heat for 10-15 minutes, until the barley is tender and has absorbed all the water.

2. Rinse with cool running water in a sieve or colander, and drain.

3. Combine the barley, salad greens, cherry tomatoes, lemon zest, juice, and onion in a bowl and toss to combine.

4. In a small mixing bowl, combine the chimichurri ingredients — parsley, coriander, chilli flakes, garlic, oil, and vinegar — and stir well.

5. Top the barley salad with beef slices, then spoon over the chimichurri to serve.

Banana-Hazelnut Smoothie

Ingredients

☐ 1 frozen medium banana (approx. 110g) or fresh banana, plus handful ice

☐ 1 cup Complete Dairy High Protein milk (250ml)

☐ 100 g low-fat Greek plain yoghurt

☐ 25 g Whole rolled oats (approx. ¼ cup)

☐ 5 roasted hazelnuts

Directions

1. Blend all of the ingredients together until smooth, then serve.

2. TIP: You may like to add a teaspoon of honey for a daily indulgence.

Cauliflower and celeriac soup

Ingredients

☐ 1 tbsp olive oil

☐ 1 onion roughly chopped

☐ 250 g celeriac peeled and roughly chopped

☐ 450 g cauliflower roughly chopped

☐ 440 g canned cannellini beans rinsed and drained

☐ 4 cups vegetable or chicken stock

☐ Flaky sea salt and freshly ground black pepper to taste

☐ Olive oil Extra virgin

Directions

1. Heat the oil in a large heavy-bottomed saucepan over medium-high heat and cook the onion for 2 to 3 minutes.

2. Add the celeriac, cauliflower, and beans and cook for another 3–4 minutes, stirring frequently.

3. Pour in the stock. Increase the heat and bring to a boil, then reduce the heat and simmer, covered, for 15–20 minutes or until the vegetables are cooked through.

4. Allow to cool slightly, then puree with an immersion blender or in a blender. Season with salt and pepper. Ladle the soup into bowls and finish with a drizzle of extra virgin olive oil.

Chai-spiced Smoothie Bowl

Ingredients

☐ ½ frozen medium banana or fresh banana, plus handful ice

☐ ¼ cup Complete Dairy High Protein milk (approx. 60ml)

☐ 200 g low fat plain Greek yoghurt

☐ 1 tsp ground cinnamon

☐ ½ tso ground ginger

☐ 3 tsp chia seeds

☐ 40 g Freedom Foods Barley + Muesli, Cranberry & Nuts

Directions

1. Blend all of the ingredients together except for the Protein 1st cereal,then pour into a bowl. The smoothie will continue to thicken over the next few minutes as chia soaks up water, so leave for 2-3 minutes and then top with the cereal. Enjoy!

2. TIP: You may like to top with a teaspoon of honey as a daily indulgences.

Cinnamon oat & almond loaf

Ingredients

☐ 50 g Ground almond meal

☐ 125 ml Low fat milk

☐ 80 g Unsalted margarine

☐ 110 g Low GI cane sugar

☐ 1 tsp Vanilla extract

☐ 2 Large eggs, lightly beaten

☐ 150 g Self-raising flour

☐ 2 tsp Ground cinnamon

☐ 22 g Rolled oats

☐ 2 Pears, peeled, cored & diced

☐ 55 g Low GI cane sugar

☐ 50 g Flaked almonds

☐ 2 tbsp Plain flour

☐ 25 g Unsalted butter, melted

Directions

1. Preheat oven to 180°C conventional or 160°C fan forced. Grease and line an 8cm x 26cm loaf pan with baking paper.

2. Combine almond meal and milk

3. Cream butter, CSR LoGiCane™ Low GI cane sugar and vanilla extract with an electric mixer until light and creamy. Add eggs gradually, beating well after each addition. Sift in flour and cinnamon, add oats and combined almond meal and milk. Pour half the mixture into prepared pan. Top with pear and cover with remaining cake batter. Sprinkle with topping.

4. Bake for 1 hour or until skewer comes out clean. Transfer to cooling rack and cool slightly, before slicing.

Chicken & herb meatball soup

Ingredients

- [ ] 60 g All-Bran® Original

- [ ] 350 g Lean chicken breast mince

- [ ] 2 Garlic cloves, crushed

- [ ] 2 tbsp Finely chopped flat-leaf parsley, plus extra to garnish

- [ ] 1 tbsp Finely chopped basil

- [ ] 1 Egg (assumed medium)

- [ ] 2 tsp Olive oil

- [ ] 1 Onion, finely chopped (assumed medium)

- [ ] 1 Carrot, peeled, diced

- [ ] 1 Stick celery, diced (assumed medium)

- [ ] 1.5 litres Salt reduced chicken stock

- [ ] 65 g Low Gi rice

- [ ] 200 g Fresh corn kernels

- [ ] 150 g Green beans, trimmed, sliced into 1cm rounds

- [ ] Finely grated lemon zest, to garnish

Directions

1. To make the meatballs, place All-Bran® Original in a food processor and process until coarse crumbs. Place the All-Bran®Original, the chicken mince, half the garlic, the parsley, basil and egg in a large bowl. Using clean hands, mix all ingredients until well combined. Using slightly wet hands, take heaped teaspoons of the mixture and roll into balls. Set aside.

2. Heat the oil in a large saucepan over a medium heat. Cook the onion, carrot and celery, stirring occasionally, for 5 minutes or until soft. Add garlic, cook for 1 minute more. Add sock, bring to the boil. Add rice, simmer for 10 minutes or until almost tender.

3. Add corn and beans, simmer for 2 minutes. Reduce the heat to low, add the meatballs in batches and simmer gently for 3-4 minutes or until just cooked through and they float on the surface.

4. Serve garnished with extra chopped parsley and grated lemon zest.

Chicken and parsley salad pitas

Ingredients

☐ 60 ml White wine vinegar

☐ 1 small red onion, finely chopped

☐ 1 tsp Dijon mustard

☐ 1 tsp Moroccan seasoning, or harissa seasoning

☐ 400 g chicken breast, lean, raw, halved horizontally

☐ 2 celery sticks, thinly sliced

☐ 1 cup parsley

☐ ½ cup fresh mint

☐ 2 medium tomatoes, chopped

☐ 4 wholemeal pita bread

☐ 80 g avocado chopped

Directions

1. Using a fork, whisk together the vinegar, onion, mustard and harissa seasoning in a large heatproof bowl. Set aside.

2. Preheat a chargrill pan over medium-high heat. Add the chicken and cook, turning once, for 8 minutes or until golden and cooked through. Transfer to a plate, cover loosely with foil and rest for 5 minutes. Thinly slice, then add to the onion mixture in the bowl, along with any resting juices on the plate.

3. Add the celery, parsley, mint and tomato to the chicken mixture and gently toss to combine. Spoon evenly onto the pita bread, top with the avocado and serve.

Barbecued chilli mint lamb and tomato salad

Ingredients

☐ 250 g Lamb fillet, trimmed

☐ Extra-virgin olive oil, for brushing

☐ 30 g Mint leaves, roughly torn

☐ 4 Small vine-ripened tomatoes, cut into eighths, or 8 cherry tomatoes, halved

☐ ½ Red capsicum (pepper), sliced into strips

☐ 1 Lebanese (short) cucumber, sliced into rounds

☐ 1 Red chilli, seeds removed and thinly sliced (optional)

☐ Freshly ground black pepper

☐ 2 tsp Extra-virgin olive oil

☐ ½ Lemon, juiced

ZESTY BULGUR WHEAT

☐ 90 g Bulgur wheat

☐ 125 ml Boiling water

☐ Finely grated zest and juice of 1 lemon

Directions

1. Lightly brush the lamb fillet with a little oil. Cook on a preheated barbecue or in a char-grill pan for 3–4 minutes each side, or until cooked to your liking. Remove the meat, wrap in foil and leave it to rest for 10 minutes.

2. Put the mint, tomatoes, capsicum, cucumber and chilli, if using, in a serving bowl. Season with pepper. Make a dressing by combining the oil and lemon juice in a screw-top jar and shake well.

3. To make the zesty bulgur wheat, put the bulgur wheat in a bowl and pour over the boiling water. Cover with foil (or plastic wrap or a plate) and leave to steam for about 15 minutes, or until the water has absorbed. Fluff up the grains with a fork and stir in the lemon zest and juice.

4. Slice the lamb fillet thinly across the grain, toss with the salad ingredients and the bulgur wheat, then pour over the dressing and toss to coat.

Chickpea curry with pumpkin and baby spinach

Ingredients

☐ 2 tbsp Extra virgin olive oil

☐ 1 Medium onion, finely chopped

☐ 2 Cloves garlic, crushed

☐ 1 tsp Chilli powder

☐ 1 tsp Ground coriander

☐ 2 tsp Ground cumin

☐ 500 g Plain tomato pasta sauce

☐ 1 ½ cups Cooked chickpeas (garbanzos)

☐ 320 g Peeled pumpkin (butternut squash), chopped into small pieces

☐ Pinch salt, optional

☐ 120 g Baby spinach leaves

☐ 2 tsp Freshly chopped coriander (cilantro)

Directions

1. Heat oil in a large saucepan and sauté onion for about 5 minutes until soft. Stir in garlic and cook for 30 seconds.

2. Mix in chilli powder, coriander, cumin, tomato pasta sauce and ½ cup of water. Stir well.

3. Add chickpeas and pumpkin pieces, and bring to boil. Adjust flavour with extra salt, if desired.

4. Reduce heat and simmer for around 15 minutes or until pumpkin is tender.

5. Stir through baby spinach leaves until they start to wilt, followed by coriander, and serve immediately.

Berry sundae

Ingredients

☐ 1 2 litre 98% Fat Free Vanilla ice cream

☐ 400 g Mixed berries (fresh or frozen)

☐ 1 Punnet of strawberries, halved

☐ ½ cup Cup soft icing mixture

☐ ¼ cup Water

☐ Brandy snap wafers or chocolate leaves for garnish

Directions

1. Combine berries in a small bowl (reserving a few for garnish) with the icing sugar and water and mix well.

2. Scoop the 98% Fat Free Vanilla ice cream into large balls and place one at the base of each serving glass

3. Drizzle over a little of the berry mixture and layer with another 2 scoops of ice cream and berry mixture.

4. Garnish with reserved berries and a brandy snap wafers or chocolate leaves.

5. Serve immediately!

Vegetable frittata

INGREDIENTS

☐ Olive oil spray

☐ 1 tablespoon olive oil

☐ 500g frozen stir-fry vegetable mix, thawed

☐ 6 eggs

☐ 125ml (1/2 cup) milk

☐ Mixed salad leaves, to serve

Directions

1. Preheat oven to 180°C. Spray a 20cm (base measurement) square cake pan with oil. Line base and

sides with non-stick baking paper, allowing the 2 long sides to overhang.

2. Heat oil in a large non-stick frying pan over medium-high heat. Stir-fry the vegetables for 3 minutes or until soft. Transfer to the prepared pan.

3. Use a balloon whisk to whisk eggs and milk in a bowl until combined. Season with salt and pepper. Pour over the vegetables. Bake for 25-30 minutes or until set and light golden.

4. Set aside for 10 minutes to cool slightly. Serve with salad leaves.

Gluten-free chicken and vegetable pie

INGREDIENTS

☐ 1 tablespoon sunflower oil

☐ 1 garlic clove, finely chopped

☐ 400g chicken breast fillets, diced

☐ 1 medium zucchini, chopped

☐ 1 medium carrot, peeled, chopped

☐ 1 medium potato, peeled, diced

☐ 2 cups Massel chicken style liquid stock

☐ 2 tablespoons gluten-free cornflour

☐ ¼ cup chopped fresh flat-leaf parsley leaves

☐ ¼ cup fresh tarragon leaves, finely chopped

GLUTEN-FREE PIE PASTRY

☐ ½ cup rice flour

☐ ½ cup gluten-free cornflour

☐ ¼ cup buckwheat flour

☐ ¼ teaspoon salt

☐ 50g Nuttelex dairy-free spread, chopped

☐ ¼ cup sunflower oil

☐ 1 egg, lightly beaten

Directions

1. Preheat oven to 200C/180C fan-forced. Heat oil in a saucepan over medium heat. Add garlic and chicken. Cook, stirring, for 5 minutes or until browned. Add zucchini, carrot and potato. Cook for 3 minutes. Add 1 cup stock to pan.

2. Place cornflour and ¼ cup remaining stock in a bowl. Stir to form a paste. Stir in remaining stock. Stir cornflour mixture into chicken mixture. Bring to the boil. Reduce heat to medium-low. Simmer for 5 minutes or until just

thickened. Stir through parsley and tarragon. Spoon mixture into a 5 cup-capacity ovenproof dish.

3. Make pastry: Sift rice flour, cornflour, buckwheat flour and salt into a large bowl. Add spread, 1 tablespoon cold water and sunflower oil. Using a flat-bladed knife, stir to form a dough, adding extra cold water if needed. Knead dough for 3 minutes or until smooth and combined. Shape dough into a disc.

4. Roll pastry out on a lightly floured surface until large enough to cover dish. Place pastry over filling. Pinch edges to seal. Brush with egg. Bake for 35 to 40 minutes or until pastry is golden. Stand for 5 minutes to cool. Serve.

Sautéed Shrimp

Ingredients

☐ 4 sun-dried tomato halves

☐ ¼ cup hot water

☐ 1 tablespoon olive oil

☐ ½ pound cooked and peeled shrimp (20–24 count size)

☐ 1 cup baby spinach leaves, rinsed and drained

☐ 1 teaspoon dried basil

☐ ¼ teaspoon black pepper

Directions

1. Place sun-dried tomato halves into a small bowl. Pour hot water over the tomatoes and set aside for 10 minutes, stirring occasionally. After 10 minutes, remove tomatoes from the water, reserving the water for later use. Chop tomatoes and set aside. In a large sauté pan, heat olive oil. Add cooked shrimp and sauté.

2. Add chopped tomato and spinach, then pour in the ¼ cup reserved hot water and continue cooking. Add dried basil and black pepper, stir until combined, and serve immediately.

Spaghetti squash with chunky tomato sauce

Ingredients

☐ 1 tablespoon extra virgin olive oil

☐ 2 cups (6 ounces) sliced baby bella mushrooms

☐ ½ cup diced onion

☐ ½ cup diced green bell pepper

☐ 1 can (about 14 ounces) no-salt-added diced tomatoes

□ ½ cup no-salt-added pasta sauce

□ 1/3 cup water

□ ½ teaspoon dried oregano

□ ¼ teaspoon salt (optional)

□ 1/8 teaspoon black pepper

□ 4 (3-ounce) cooked chicken sausage links, cut into pieces

□ 1 spaghetti squash (about 4 pounds)

□ 2 tablespoons chopped fresh Italian parsley

Directions

1. Cut spaghetti squash lengthwise in half. Remove seeds. Place squash in 12×8-inch microwavable dish. Cover with vented plastic wrap. Microwave on high 9 minutes or until squash separates easily into strands when tested with fork. Cut each squash half lengthwise in half; separate strands with fork.

2. Heat oil in large skillet over medium-high heat. Add mushrooms, onion, and bell pepper; cook and stir 7 minutes or until vegetables are tender.

3. Stir tomatoes, pasta sauce, water, oregano, salt, if desired, and black pepper into skillet. Cover bring to a

simmer; reduce heat and simmer 5 minutes. Stir sausage pieces into sauce.

4. Divide squash evenly among 4 plates. Spoon sauce over squash; sprinkle with parsley.

Savory Pumpkin Hummus

Ingredients

☐ 1 can (15 ounces) solid-pack pumpkin

☐ 3 tablespoons chopped fresh parsley, plus additional for garnish

☐ 3 tablespoons tahini

☐ 3 tablespoons fresh lemon juice

☐ 3 cloves garlic

☐ 1 teaspoon ground cumin

☐ ½ teaspoon salt

☐ 1/8 teaspoon black pepper

☐ 1/8 teaspoon ground red pepper, plus additional for garnish

☐ Assorted vegetable sticks

Directions

1. Combine pumpkin, 3 tablespoons parsley, tahini, lemon juice, garlic, cumin, salt, black pepper, and 1/8 teaspoon ground red pepper in food processor or blender; process until smooth. Cover and refrigerate at least 2 hours to allow flavors to develop.

2. Sprinkle with additional ground red pepper, if desired. Garnish with additional parsley. Serve with assorted vegetable sticks.

Mediterranean Deviled Eggs

Ingredients

☐ ¼ cup finely diced cucumber

☐ ¼ cup finely diced tomato

☐ 2 teaspoons fresh lemon juice

☐ 1/8 teaspoon salt

☐ 6 hard-cooked eggs, peeled and sliced in half lengthwise

☐ 1/3 cup roasted garlic or any flavor hummus

☐ Chopped fresh parsley (optional)

Directions

1. Combine cucumber, tomato, lemon juice, and salt in small bowl; gently mix.

2. Remove yolks from eggs; discard. Spoon 1 heaping teaspoon hummus into each egg half. Top with ½ teaspoon cucumber–tomato mixture and parsley, if desired. Serve immediately.

Maple and Apple Pork Chops

Ingredients

☐ Nonstick cooking spray

☐ 4 boneless pork chops (about 1 pound)

☐ 2 small apples (2–2 ½ inches in diameter)

☐ 1/8 cup lite, maple-flavored syrup

☐ 1/8 cup water

Directions

1. Spray large skillet with nonstick cooking spray. Heat over medium heat, then add pork chops to pan so that they are not touching each other. Brown pork chops on both sides, approximately 2 minutes on each side. Core apples (leaving skin on), then dice to yield

approximately 1 ½ cups. Sprinkle apples into hot skillet. In a small bowl, combine maple-flavored syrup and water and stir until well combined.

2. Pour liquid into skillet, and cover. Cook approximately 5–7 minutes on medium heat until pork chops are cooked through and internal temperature is 160°F.

Basil chicken bites

Ingredients

☐ 1 pound chicken breast tenderloins

☐ 1 ½ teaspoons dried basil

☐ ¼ teaspoon black pepper

☐ 1/8 teaspoon salt (optional)

☐ ¼ teaspoon garlic powder

☐ 1 tablespoon extra-virgin olive oil

Directions

1. Cut tenderloins into bite-size pieces, about 2 inches long. Place pieces in a plastic bag along with basil, pepper, salt, and garlic powder. Shake well to coat. Heat olive oil in a large skillet over medium heat. Add chicken.

2. Sauté over medium heat, turning frequently, until chicken is cooked through, about 10–12 minutes.

Spanish Paella with Shrimp and Scallops

Ingredients

☐ 1 tablespoon olive oil

☐ 2 cloves garlic, minced

☐ 2 cups chopped onions

☐ 1 cup short-grain white rice

☐ 1 cup low-sodium chicken broth

☐ ½ cup dry white wine

☐ ½ cup water

☐ 1 ½ tablespoons fresh-squeezed lemon juice

☐ ½ teaspoon paprika

☐ ½ teaspoon saffron

☐ ¼ cup boiling water

☐ 4 small plum tomatoes, chopped

☐ ¼ cup chopped fresh parsley

□ 1 jar (4 ounces) roasted red peppers, drained and chopped

□ ½ cup frozen peas, defrosted

□ 10 large scallops

□ 20 large shrimp, shelled and cleaned

Directions

1. Heat olive oil in a large skillet or sauté pan. Add garlic, onions, and rice and cook, stirring, for 5 minutes. Stir in broth, wine, water, lemon juice, and paprika. Stir saffron into boiling water and add to mixture. Stir in tomatoes, parsley, and roasted red peppers.

2. Cook uncovered for approximately 10 minutes on medium-low heat, stirring occasionally. Stir in peas, scallops, and shrimp and cook for additional 7–10 minutes until scallops and shrimp are done and rice is tender. Serve immediately.

Stuffed pork tenderloin with collard greens

Ingredients

□ 1 pound lean pork tenderloin

☐ 12 dried apricot halves (about ½ cup)

☐ 1 teaspoon black pepper

☐ 1 teaspoon onion powder

☐ 1 teaspoon oregano

☐ 1 pound collard greens, stemmed, washed, and drained, but not dry

☐ 1 tablespoon extra-virgin olive oil

☐ ¾ cup diced onion

☐ 1 clove garlic, minced

☐ 2 dashes salt

Directions

1. Heat oven to 400°F. Line a baking pan with nonstick aluminum foil (or use regular aluminum foil sprayed with nonfat cooking spray). Place tenderloin on a cutting board, and use a slightly oiled (olive oil) sharpening steel or boning knife to make a hole in the center of the tenderloin all the way through. Stuff dried apricots into the cavity, working from one end at a time and making sure to stuff them all the way into the middle.

2. Place tenderloin in pan and sprinkle with black pepper, onion powder, and oregano. Cook for 45 minutes, or until a meat thermometer reads at least

160°F. If you prefer your pork well done, cook until thermometer reads 170°F. Remove and let rest 5 minutes before slicing.

3. While meat is resting, roll a collard leaf into a tight roll. Using a sharp slicing knife, slice into thin strips. Repeat until all of the greens resemble green ribbons. Heat oil in a large skillet over medium-high heat and add onion and garlic. Cook until onions are almost transparent. Add greens (which should still be damp) and sauté, moving rapidly until greens have relaxed and deepened in color, 2–3 minutes. If mixture starts to stick to the pan, add 1 tablespoon water. Remove greens from heat.

4. To serve, place approximately 1 cup of greens on a dinner plate. Cut tenderloin into 1 ½-inch slices. Place meat slices on top of greens.

Grilled Salmon Fillet with Chili-Infused Blackberry Sauce

Ingredients

☐ 4 four-ounce salmon fillets (or steaks)

☐ 1 cup fresh blackberries, washed and drained

☐ ¼ cup unsweetened white grape juice

☐ 1 tablespoon fresh lemon juice

☐ 1 tablespoon honey

☐ 1 tablespoon extra-virgin olive oil

☐ 1 tablespoon sweet Chinese chili sauce

Directions

1. Heat gas or wood grill. Grill salmon fillets on hot grill until they reach desired doneness. (For well-done, grill for approximately 4–5 minutes on each side for 1-inch-thick fish).

2. Sauce: In a food processor or blender, combine sauce ingredients and blend until smooth. To serve, top each cooked fillet with 3 tablespoons of sauce

Sesame-Ginger Grilled Salmon

Ingredients

☐ 1 tablespoon reduced-sodium soy sauce

☐ ¼ cup fresh-squeezed orange juice (for best flavor)

☐ 1 tablespoon horseradish mustard

☐ 2 dashes cayenne pepper

☐ ½ teaspoon ground ginger

☐ 1 teaspoon minced garlic

☐ 1 tablespoon honey

☐ 4 boneless salmon fillets (3 ounces each)

☐ 1 teaspoon toasted sesame seeds

Directions

1. In a small bowl, whisk together soy sauce, orange juice, mustard, cayenne pepper, ginger, garlic, and honey. Place salmon fillets in a large zip-top bag and drizzle evenly with marinade. Seal bag and shake gently to coat fish. Marinate in the refrigerator for 1 hour, turning occasionally.

2. Preheat grill to medium-high heat (around 350°F). Place salmon on the grill, reserving marinade. Baste fish with marinade, then grill about 6 minutes on each side, or until fish flakes easily when pierced with a fork. Bring remaining marinade to a boil and boil 2–3 minutes. (Do not use remaining marinade unless it is boiled). Drizzle cooked salmon with heated marinade and top with toasted sesame seeds.

Grilled Romaine and Asparagus Salad

Ingredients

☐ 1 six-ounce head romaine lettuce

☐ Nonstick cooking spray

☐ Aluminum foil

☐ 4 medium spears or 8 thin spears fresh asparagus

☐ ¼ cup thinly sliced red onion

☐ 12 grape tomatoes

☐ 1 tablespoon shredded Parmesan cheese

☐ ¼ cup fat-free Italian salad dressing

Directions

1. Heat grill. Cut lettuce head lengthwise in half, but do not trim off the base holding the leaves together; wash lettuce and pat dry. Spray a 12-inch piece of foil (or a larger piece, if needed) with nonstick cooking spray. Place lettuce halves on foil and place on hot grill. Grill each side of halves for 2 minutes until slightly browned. Remove from grill and cool.

2. Cut off base, then slice lettuce horizontally into ribbons, about 1 inch wide. While grill is still hot, grill asparagus on same foil, turning constantly, until slightly

browned. Slice asparagus diagonally into 1-inch pieces. Place lettuce and asparagus in a medium salad bowl along with sliced onion, tomatoes, and Parmesan cheese. Toss, add dressing, then toss again.

Pineapple Ginger Glazed Baked Salmon

Ingredients

☐ 1 ½ lbs salmon, cut into individual fillets

☐ 3 Tbsp avocado oil

☐ ½ cup pineapple juice

☐ 1 ½ inch nub fresh ginger, peeled

☐ 2 cloves garlic

☐ ½ tsp sea salt

☐ 2 Tbsp coconut aminos, or liquid aminos, optional

Directions

1. Add all of the ingredients for the marinade to a blender and blend until smooth. Place salmon fillets into a zip lock bag or sealable container and pour marinade over the fish. Seal and move the fish around until everything is well-coated in marinade. Refrigerate at least 1 hour (up to 8).

2. When you're ready to bake, preheat the oven to 350 degrees F. Place the salmon in a casserole dish, along with the marinade. Bake for 20 to 30 minutes, until fish is cooked through.

3. Spoon the marinade over the fish (it will have thickened during the baking process) before serving and serve with choice of side dishes.

Vegetable and Sausage Skillet

Ingredients

☐ 1.5Tbsp avocado oil

☐ 1 (12-oz.) package pre-cooked sausage of choice, sliced

☐ 4 large carrots, sliced

☐ 2 medium zucchini, chopped

☐ 1 large red bell bell pepper, chopped

☐ 2 tsp dried parsley

☐ ½ tsp sea salt

Directions

1. Heat the avocado oil in a large skillet over medium-high heat.

2. Add the sliced sausage and brown for 2 to 3 minutes, or until sausage begins to get some color and a crispy char.

3. Add the chopped carrots, zucchini and bell pepper and stir well. Cover skillet and cook until carrots begin to soften, about 5 minutes. Remove the cover and stir in the parsley and sea salt. Continue cooking until vegetables reach desired done-ness, about another 5 minutes.

4. Serve as is or with choice of side dishes. I like eating mine over a bed of steamed rice!

Layered chicken, lemon and risoni bake

INGREDIENTS

☐ 4 garlic cloves, crushed

☐ 1 teaspoon ground cumin

☐ 1 teaspoon paprika

☐ ½ teaspoon dried chilli flakes

☐ 2 tablespoons preserved lemon rind, finely chopped

☐ 6 chicken thigh fillets, trimmed, halved

☐ ¼ teaspoon saffron threads

☐ ¾ cup water, boiling

☐ 1 tablespoon extra virgin olive oil

☐ 2 brown onions, halved, thinly sliced

☐ ¾ cup dried risoni

☐ 1 cup Massel salt reduced chicken style liquid stock

☐ 1/3 cup pitted Sicilian green olives, quartered

☐ ¼ cup fresh coriander leaves

Directions

1. Combine garlic, cumin, paprika, chilli and ½ the preserved lemon rind in a large glass or ceramic bowl. Add chicken. Toss to coat. Cover. Refrigerate overnight to marinate, if time permits.

2. Preheat oven to 180C/160C fan-forced. Place saffron and boiling water in a small heatproof bowl.

3. Heat oil in a 6cm-deep, 22cm x 30cm (base) flameproof roasting pan over medium-high heat. Cook chicken, turning, for 5 minutes or until browned all over. Transfer to a plate.

4. Reduce heat to medium. Add onion to pan. Cook, stirring occasionally, for 10 minutes or until softened and slightly caramelised. Add saffron mixture, risoni and stock. Season with salt and pepper. Stir to combine. Arrange chicken on risoni mixture. Bring to the boil.

Cover pan with lid or tightly with foil to prevent steam escaping. Carefully transfer pan to oven.

5. Bake for 25 to 30 minutes or until stock is absorbed and risoni is tender. Sprinkle with olives, coriander and remaining preserved lemon rind. Serve.

Masala egg curry

INGREDIENTS

☐ 6 eggs, at room temperature

☐ 2 tablespoons vegetable oil

☐ 1 large red onion, halved, thinly sliced

☐ ½ teaspoon ground turmeric

☐ ½ teaspoon chilli powder

☐ 4cm piece fresh ginger, finely grated

☐ 1 long green chilli, thinly sliced

☐ 270ml can coconut milk

☐ 150g green beans, trimmed

☐ 150g sugar snap peas, trimmed

☐ ½ teaspoon garam masala, toasted

☐ ½ cup fresh coriander leaves

☐ Steamed basmati rice, to serve

Directions

1. Place eggs in a saucepan. Cover with cold water. Bring to the boil over high heat, stirring occasionally. Reduce heat to medium. Simmer for 3 minutes. Remove pan from heat. Carefully, transfer eggs to a board. Set aside to cool slightly.

2. Meanwhile, heat oil in large saucepan over medium heat. Cook onion, stirring, for 7 minutes or until light golden. Add turmeric, chilli powder, ginger and 1/2 the green chilli. Cook, stirring, for 1 minute or until fragrant.

3. Add coconut milk and ½ cup water. Bring to the boil. Reduce heat to low. Simmer for 5 minutes or until liquid reduces by half.

4. Peel eggs. Add beans, peas and eggs to curry. Cook, stirring, for 1 to 2 minutes or until beans are just tender and eggs are heated through. Cut eggs in half. Sprinkle curry with garam masala, coriander and remaining chilli and serve with rice.

Salsa verde chicken with ricotta-stuffed capsicum

INGREDIENTS

- ☐ 100g reduced-fat fresh ricotta, crumbled
- ☐ 4 baby red capsicum
- ☐ 1 ½ tablespoons extra virgin olive oil
- ☐ 4 x 150g chicken breast fillets, trimmed
- ☐ Cooked risoni, to serve
- ☐ Salad leaves, to serve

SALSA VERDE

- ☐ ¾ cup finely chopped fresh flat-leaf parsley leaves
- ☐ 1/3 cup finely chopped fresh basil leaves, plus extra to serve
- ☐ ½ red onion, finely chopped
- ☐ 1 tablespoon wholegrain mustard
- ☐ 2 tablespoons lemon juice
- ☐ 1 garlic clove, crushed
- ☐ ¼ cup extra virgin olive oil

Directions

1. Make Salsa Verde: Combine parsley, basil, onion, mustard, lemon juice, garlic and oil in a bowl. Season with salt and pepper.

2. Place half the Salsa Verde in a bowl. Add ricotta. Mix well. Cut tops from capsicum and reserve. Using a teaspoon, scoop out and discard seeds. Spoon ricotta mixture evenly among capsicum. Drizzle with 1/2 the oil.

3. Rub remaining oil over chicken. Season with salt and pepper. Heat a barbecue grill on medium-high heat. Cook chicken for 4 to 5 minutes each side or until browned and cooked through. Remove from heat. Slice chicken.

4. Cook stuffed capsicum and tops on grill for 2 to 3 minutes each side or until lightly charred and heated through. Place tops on capsicum.

5. Serve chicken with capsicum, risoni, salad leaves, remaining Salsa Verde and extra basil leaves.

Cottage cheese and salad sandwich

Ingredients

☐ 200 g cottage cheese

☐ 50 g grated cheddar cheese

☐ Shredded spinach leaves

☐ Green onion, thinly sliced

☐ Toasted sesame seeds

☐ Lemon juice

☐ Grated carrot

☐ Original Bread

Directions

1. Mix together cottage cheese, cheddar cheese, spinach, onion, sesame seeds and a little lemon juice. Spread over bread and top with carrot, and lettuce.

Crisp-skinned salmon

Ingredients

☐ 4 pieces salmon, about 180g/6oz each (middle section is best)

☐ 1 tbsp olive oil

☐ Sea or kosher salt

Directions

1. Pat the fish dry with kitchen paper.

2. Heat the oil in a non-stick frying pan over moderate heat.

3. Salt the skin of the fish with salt and place skin-side down in the pan and cook until golden and crispy. This can take 5–8 minutes depending on the size and thickness of the fish pieces. By the time the skin is crisp, the fish is almost cooked.

4. Turn the fish over carefully, then remove from the pan and allow to rest uncovered (not on its skin side) for three minutes. The residual heat will finish cooking it perfectly.

5. Serve with plenty of veggies or salad following our healthy plate plan.

Apple bircher muesli

Ingredients

☐ 2 cups rolled oats

☐ 1 cup milk

☐ ¾ cup creamy natural yogurt

☐ 2 lemons, juiced

☐ 3 apples

☐ 2 tbsp sultanas

☐ 2 tbsp dried pears, chopped

☐ 2 tbsp roasted hazelnuts, roughly chopped

☐ 1 tbsp pepitas

☐ 2 tsp sunflower seeds

☐ 2 tsp sesame seeds

☐ Honey to taste

Directions

1. Place the oats in a large bowl and stir through the milk and yogurt. Take 2 of the apples, cut into quarters and leaving the skin on, coarsely grate. Toss in the lemon juice and stir into the oat mixture.

2. Stir through the sultanas and dried pears. When ready to serve scatter over the hazelnuts, pepitas and sesame seeds. Divide among 4 bowls. Slice the remaining apples and put on top. Drizzle with honey to taste.

Asian-style Pearl Couscous with grilled salmon

Ingredients

- [ ] 2 tbsp olive oil

- [ ] 1 tsp curry powder

- [ ] 1 tsp chilli paste

- [ ] 4 salmon fillets, each about 125g

- [ ] ½ brown onion, finely chopped

- [ ] 1½ cups Pearl Couscous

- [ ] 2½ cups hot strong chicken stock (low or reduced salt)

- [ ] Freshly ground black pepper

- [ ] 2 cups cleaned bean shoots

- [ ] 2 cups baby spinach leaves

- [ ] 4 spring onions, cut into small pieces

- [ ] ½ cup coriander leaves

- [ ] 4 quarters of lime or lemon

Directions

1. In a small bowl mix oil, curry powder and chilli paste.

2. Very lightly brush salmon fillets with half the spicy oil.

3. Place remaining spicy oil in a non-stick pan with onion and cook on medium heat while stirring, for 3 minutes. Add Pearl Couscous, stir well and add hot chicken stock. Bring to a simmer, cover with a lid and cook on low heat for about 8 minutes. Season with pepper to taste and stir in bean shoots and spinach leaves. Stir again and cook for a further 2 minutes until couscous is done.

4. Place salmon on a hot grill plate and cook for about 3 minutes on each side.

5. Spoon Pearl Couscous onto plates and top with salmon fillets. Sprinkle with spring onions and coriander leaves and serve with lime quarters.

Curried Pearl Couscous with

pomegranates

Ingredients

☐ 1 tbsp olive oil

☐ 250 g Blu gourmet Pearl Couscous

☐ 1 ½ cups hot vegetable or chicken stock or water

☐ ½ tsp keens curry powder

☐ ½ medium slightly firm avocado diced

☐ ½ cup pomegranate seeds

☐ 1 small dried shallot halved and sliced

☐ 4 tbsp fresh mint chopped

☐ 4 tbsp fresh parsley chopped

☐ ¼ cup toasted slivered almonds

DRESSING:

☐ 2 tbsp lemon juice

☐ 1 tsp lemon zest

☐ 1 tbsp white balsamic vinegar

☐ 2 tbsp olive oil

☐ ¼ tsp ground fresh pepper

Directions

1. Add olive oil, curry and couscous to saucepan, and stir fry for a couple of minutes on medium heat to toast the couscous and release the flavour of the curry. Add stock and simmer covered on medium heat for approximately 8 minutes or until liquid is absorbed. Remove from heat and toss into a salad bowl with the dressing and mix until cooled.

2. Add shallots, pomegranate seeds, avocado, mint and parsley and stir through gently to combine.

3. Sprinkle with toasted almonds and serve.

Fresh kale, avocado and pomegranate salad

Ingredients

☐ 300 g Curly kale leaves stripped from their stem

☐ ¼ cup Lemon juice (about 1 juiced lemon)

☐ 3 tbsp Extra virgin olive oil

☐ ½ tsp Salt

☐ 1 Avocado, cut into small cubes

☐ ½ cup Pomegranate seeds

Directions

1. Wash kale leaves thoroughly, in several changes of water. Press down firmly or use a salad spinner to remove excess water.

2. Roll up leaves and shred very finely, then transfer to a large salad bowl.

3. Add lemon juice, oil and salt, and massage well with a clean hand for a few minutes until kale softens. Allow to sit for at least 30 minutes for flavour to develop.

4. Prior to serving, fold in avocado and pomegranate seeds. Salad will keep in fridge for up to 2 days. Recipe is unsuitable for freezing.

Asparagus, **corn and brazil nut salad**

Ingredients

☐ 2 cups Low GI Brown Rice

☐ 1 bunch Asparagus, trimmed and sliced

☐ 125 g Baby corn, halved

☐ 5 Radishes, trimmed and thinly sliced

☐ 2 Green onions, trimmed and sliced

☐ 1 cup Coarsely chopped mint leaves, plus whole leaves to garnish

☐ ¾ cup Brazil nuts, toasted and roughly chopped

☐ ½ cup Pomegranate seeds

☐ ¼ cup Olive oil

☐ 2 tbsp Lemon juice

☐ 1 tbsp Dijon mustard

Directions

1. Cook the rice according to directions on the packet. Cool.

2. Cook asparagus and corn in boiling water for 2 minutes or until just tender. Rinse under cold water. Drain.

3. Add asparagus, corn, radishes, green onions, mint and ½ each of the of the brazil nuts and pomegranate seeds to rice. Combine oil, lemon juice and mustard and add to rice mixture. Toss to combine.

4. Serve salad topped with whole mint leaves, remaining chopped brazil nuts and pomegranate seeds.

Avocado & Cottage Cheese Whip on Toast

Ingredients

☐ 1 slice Burgen bread, any type, toasted

☐ 20 g avocado, mashed (approx. 1 tbsp)

☐ 160 g low-fat cottage cheese

☐ 1 ½ medium tomatoes, thickly sliced

☐ 1 tbsp fresh chives, chopped

☐ ¼ lemon, juice and zest

☐ Pinch chilli flakes

☐ Black pepper, to taste (optional)

Directions

1. Spread the avocado over the toast, sprinkle over the chilli flakes, and then arrange the tomato slices.

2. Use a bullet or small handheld blender to process the cottage cheese,lemon juice, and zest until smooth. Alternatively, this can also be done in a bowl with a fork.

3. Taste, and season with pepper if you'd like. Pour into a small bowl, top with chives. To serve, spoon the cottage cheese over the toast.

Turmeric Ginger Ground Turkey Bowls

Ingredients

For the Turmeric Ground Turkey:

☐ 3 Tbsp avocado oil

☐ ½ cup yellow onion, finely chopped

☐ 1 lb lean ground turkey

☐ 3 cloves garlic, minced

☐ 1 Tbsp fresh ginger, peeled and grated or sliced

☐ ½ tsp ground turmeric, or 2 tsp fresh turmeric, grated

☐ ½ tsp sea salt, to taste

☐ 4 stalks green onion, chopped

For the Bowls:

☐ 1 Tbsp avocado oil

☐ 2 large carrots, peeled and chopped

☐ 1 large yellow squash, chopped

☐ 1 large crown broccoli, chopped

Directions

Make the Turkey:

1. Heat the avocado oil in a large non-stick skillet over medium-high heat. Add the onion and saute, stirring occasionally, until translucent, about 3 minutes. Add the turkey and brown for 3 minutes per side before using a spatula to break it into smaller pieces. Add the remaining ingredients and stir well. Cook 5 to 8 minutes longer, or until turkey is cooked through. If desired, add any sauces, such as teriyaki sauce, coconut aminos, etc.

Saute the Vegetables:

1. You can either cook the vegetables in the same skillet as the turkey, or cook them separately. To cook them with the turkey, simply add the vegetables after browning the turkey, stir well, and cover with a lid. Cook, stirring occasionally, until vegetables reach desired done-ness and turkey is cooked through, about 8 to 12 minutes.

2. To cook the vegetables separately, heat avocado oil in a separate non-stick skillet over medium-high and add the chopped vegetables. Cover and cook 3 minutes. Remove cover and continue cooking until vegetables reach desired done-ness.

Compile the Bowls:

1. Fill bowls with desired amount of turmeric ground turkey and vegetables. If desired, you can serve over a bed of steamed brown or white rice, and/or drizzle on any of your favorite sauces.

Paleo Banana Bread

Ingredients

□ 3 large ripe bananas, mashed (1 ½ cups)

□ 2 eggs

□ 2 tsp pure vanilla extract, optional

☐ 2 Tbsp pure maple syrup

☐ 2 cups Super Fine Almond Flour

☐ 5 Tbsp tapioca flour

☐ 1 ½ tsp baking powder

☐ ¼ tsp sea salt

☐ 2 tsp ground cinnamon, optional

☐ ¼ tsp ground nutmeg, optional

Directions

1. Preheat the oven to 350 degrees F and line a 9" x 5" loaf pan with parchment paper.

2. Add all of the ingredients for the banana bread to a blender. Blend until completely smooth, but be very careful not to over-blend. (Note: If you prefer using a mixing bowl over a blender, simply mash the bananas in a mixing bowl, whisk in the eggs and pure maple syrup, then proceed to mix in the remaining ingredients.)

3. Pour banana bread batter into the prepared loaf pan and use a spoon or spatula to spread the batter into an even layer.

4. Bake for 50 to 55 minutes on the center rack of the preheated oven, until the edges of the bread are golden-

brown. Turn off the oven and allow bread to sit in the still-warm oven another 10 minutes.

5. Allow bread to cool for 30 minutes before releasing it from the loaf pan and cutting into slices.

6. Cut thick slices of bread and enjoy!

Salmon With Cilantro-Lime Salsa

Ingredients

Salmon

☐ 6-8 ounces skin-on salmon (2 fillets)

☐ ¼ teaspoon each kosher salt and pepper (mixed together)

☐ ½ teaspoon each chili powder, garlic powder and paprika (mixed together)

☐ 1 tablespoon of olive oil

Cilantro-Lime Salsa

☐ 1 tablespoon of chopped cilantro

☐ ½ teaspoon of lime juice

☐ ½ teaspoon garlic clove

☐ ¼ cup of quartered cherry tomatoes

☐ 1 tablespoon of diced red onion

☐ ½ tablespoon of olive oil

☐ Salt and pepper to taste

Directions

1. Combine first six ingredients for Cilantro-Lime Salsa in a bowl. Add salt and pepper mixture to taste. Set aside or place in the refrigerator until ready to use.

2. Pat the salmon skin dry with a paper towel. This step is necessary for a nice, crispy skin. Season the skin with half of your salt and pepper mix.

3. Season the flesh side of the salmon with the salt and pepper mix and the chili powder, garlic powder and paprika mix.

4. Heat 1 tablespoon of olive oil in a skillet over medium-high heat.

5. Once the oil is shimmering, place the salmon skin-side down; hold down for 10 to 15 seconds until it relaxes and lies flat.

6. Cook for about 5 minutes over medium-high heat before flipping over. If you feel resistance as you try to flip the salmon, let it cook a couple of minutes longer. Tip: You should be able to slide the spatula relatively easily under the fish when getting ready to flip it.

7. Turn down the heat, flip to the flesh side and let it cook over medium heat for about 3 to 5 minutes, until golden brown. Depending on the thickness of the salmon, you may want to cook it a little longer or less.

8. The fish should be opaque (pink) when done. Test for doneness by slightly cutting open the thickest part of the salmon. If it flakes, you're done!

9. Serve the salmon topped with the Cilantro-Lime Salsa and your choice of side.

Salmon Seaweed Wraps

Ingredients

☐ 1 6-ounce can salmon, drained

☐ ½ avocado, ripe when soft to the touch

☐ ½ cup celery (or 1 stalk), diced small

☐ ½ cup daikon radish (or a 3-inch piece), diced small

☐ 2 teaspoons lemon juice

☐ ¼ teaspoon salt

☐ Pepper to taste

☐ 3 nori sheets (typically used to make sushi)

☐ 3 romaine lettuce leaves, whole

☐ ½ cup cucumber, diced small

☐ ½ cup red pepper (about ½ a pepper), thinly sliced into 2-inch strips

Directions

1. In a large bowl, mash salmon, including the bones, with a fork. Scoop avocado out of the skin with a spoon and add to the salmon. Continue to mash.

2. Mix in diced celery and daikon. Add lemon juice, salt and pepper to taste. Blend well.

3. Place one nori sheet on a flat plate or cutting board. Place one romaine lettuce leaf on top of the nori sheet close to one of the edges.

4. Scoop 1/3 cup of the salmon salad mixture and spread it evenly across the length of the lettuce leaf. Top with diced cucumbers and red pepper sticks.

5. Using your hands, tightly roll the nori sheet around the lettuce and filling. Seal the wrap by dampening the edge of the nori with a little water.

Roasted Dijon Lamb With Herbs and Country Vegetables

Ingredients

☐ 20 cloves garlic, peeled (about 2 medium heads)

☐ ¼ cup Dijon mustard

☐ 2 tablespoons water

☐ 2 tablespoons fresh rosemary leaves

☐ 1 tablespoon fresh thyme

☐ 1 ¼ teaspoons salt, divided

☐ 1 teaspoon black pepper

☐ Nonstick cooking spray

☐ 4 ½ pounds boneless leg of lamb, trimmed

☐ 1 pound parsnips, cut diagonally into ½-inch pieces

☐ 1 pound carrots, cut diagonally into ½-inch pieces

☐ 2 large onions, cut into ½-inch wedges

☐ 3 tablespoons extra-virgin olive oil, divided

Directions

1. Combine garlic, mustard, water, rosemary, thyme, ¾ teaspoon salt and pepper in food processor; process until

smooth. Spoon mixture over top and sides of lamb. Cover and refrigerate at least 8 hours.

2. Preheat oven to 500°F. Line broiler pan with foil; top with broiler rack. Coat rack with nonstick cooking spray. Combine parsnips, carrots, onions and 2 tablespoons oil in large bowl; toss to coat. Spread evenly on broiler rack; top with lamb.

3. Roast 15 minutes. Reduce oven temperature to 325°F. Roast 1 hour 20 minutes, or until internal temperature reaches 155°F for medium or to desired doneness.

4. Remove lamb to cutting board; let stand 10 minutes before slicing. Continue roasting vegetables 10 minutes.

5. Transfer vegetables to large bowl. Add remaining 1 tablespoon oil and ½ teaspoon salt; toss to coat. Thinly slice lamb and serve with vegetables.

Fajita-Seasoned Grilled Chicken

Ingredients

☐ 2 boneless skinless chicken breasts (about 4 ounces each)

☐ 1 bunch green onions, ends trimmed

☐ 1 tablespoon olive oil

☐ 2 teaspoons fajita seasoning mix

Directions

1. Prepare grill for direct cooking.

2. Brush chicken and green onions with oil. Sprinkle both sides of chicken breasts with seasoning mix. Grill chicken and onions 6 to 8 minutes or until chicken is no longer pink in center.

3. Serve chicken with onions.

Grilled Salmon Salad

Ingredients

☐ 1/3 cup plus 2 tablespoons fat-free raspberry or balsamic vinaigrette salad dressing, divided

☐ 4 skinless salmon fillets (about ¼ pound and ¾ inch thick)

☐ ½ teaspoon black pepper

☐ ¼ teaspoon salt

☐ 8 cups spring mix salad greens

☐ 2 cups cherry tomatoes, halved

☐ ¼ cup fresh basil, chopped (optional)

Directions

1. Prepare grill for direct cooking. Brush 2 tablespoons dressing over salmon fillets. Sprinkle with pepper and salt. Grill salmon on covered grill over medium-high heat 5 to 6 minutes, or until center is opaque.

2. Combine greens, tomatoes and remaining 1/3 cup dressing in large bowl; toss gently. Transfer to 4 plates. Top with salmon; sprinkle with basil, if desired.

3. Note: To broil the salmon, preheat broiler. Place salmon on an oiled broiler pan. Broil 4 inches from heat 6 to 7 minutes or just until the salmon begins to flake when tested with a fork.

Spiced Citrus Tea

Ingredients

☐ 1 Spiced Citrus Tea bag

☐ Boiling water

☐ 1 to 2 teaspoons orange juice

☐ Honey (optional)

☐ Orange slices (optional)

Directions

1. Place tea bag in cup or mug. Pour boiling water over tea bag; steep 3 to 5 minutes. Remove tea bag, pressing out liquid. Discard tea bag. Serve with orange juice and honey, if desired. Garnish with orange slices.

Avocado Salsa

Ingredients

☐ 1 medium avocado, peeled, cored and diced

☐ 1 cup chopped onion

☐ 1 cup peeled seeded chopped cucumber

☐ 1 Anaheim pepper, seeded and chopped

☐ ½ cup chopped fresh tomato

☐ 2 tablespoons chopped fresh cilantro, plus additional for garnish

☐ ½ teaspoon salt

☐ ¼ teaspoon hot pepper sauce

Directions

1. Combine avocado, onion, cucumber, Anaheim pepper, tomato, 2 tablespoons cilantro, salt and hot pepper sauce

into a medium bowl and gently mix. Cover and refrigerate at least 1 hour before serving. Garnish with additional cilantro.

Balsamic Grilled Pork Chops

Ingredients

☐ 2 tablespoons balsamic vinegar

☐ 2 tablespoons reduced-sodium soy sauce

☐ 1 teaspoon Dijon mustard

☐ 2 teaspoons sugar

☐ 1/8 teaspoon red pepper flakes

☐ 2 boneless pork chops, trimmed of fat (8 ounces total)

Directions

1. Combine vinegar, soy sauce, mustard, sugar, and red pepper flakes in small bowl. Stir until well blended. Reserve 1 tablespoon marinade; refrigerate until needed.

2. Place pork in large resealable food storage bag. Pour remaining over pork. Seal bag; turn to coat. Refrigerate 2 hours or up to 24 hours.

3. Spray grill pan with nonstick cooking spray; heat over medium-high heat. Remove pork from marinade;

discard marinade. Cook pork 4 minutes on each side or until just slightly pink in center. Place on plates; top with reserved 1 tablespoon marinade.

Lemon Pepper Chicken Wings

Ingredients

☐ Large baking sheet, lined with foil, with a wire rack set on top

☐ 2 pounds free-range chicken wings

☐ 2 tablespoons grated lemon zest

☐ 2 tablespoons freshly squeezed lemon juice

☐ 1 tablespoon freshly ground black pepper

☐ 1 teaspoon sea salt

Directions

1. Preheat oven to 375°F (190°C).

2. Pat chicken dry with paper towels, removing as much moisture as you can. Arrange on the wire rack over the prepared baking sheet, leaving space in between, if possible.

3. Roast in preheated oven for 30 to 35 minutes, flipping them over halfway through, until juices run clear when chicken is pierced.

4. Meanwhile, in a large bowl, combine lemon zest, lemon juice, pepper, and salt. Add wings to the lemon sauce and toss until evenly coated. Serve hot.

Rainbow Roots Slaw with Tahini Parsley Dressing

Ingredients

Tahini Parsley Dressing

☐ 1 small clove garlic, minced

☐ ¼ cup minced fresh flat-leaf (Italian) parsley

☐ 1 teaspoon ground cumin

☐ ¼ teaspoon sea salt

☐ ¼ cup tahini

☐ 2 tablespoon freshly squeezed lime juice

☐ 1 tablespoon extra virgin olive oil

☐ 2 tablespoons filtered water (approx.)

Rainbow Roots Slaw

☐ 2 cups shredded green cabbage

☐ 2 large carrots, grated

☐ 1 firm pear (such as Bosc), grated

☐ 2 medium red beets, peeled and grated

Directions

1. Dressing: In a small bowl, whisk together garlic, parsley, cumin, salt, tahini, lime juice, and oil. Whisk in 1 tablespoon water. If the dressing is too thick, add the remaining water (or more, as needed).

2. Slaw: In a large bowl, toss together cabbage, carrots, and pear. Add dressing and toss until vegetables are well coated. Add beets and toss to coat.

Broccoli Italian Style

Ingredients

☐ 1 ¼ pounds fresh broccoli

☐ 2 tablespoons lemon juice

☐ 1 teaspoon extra virgin olive oil

☐ 1 clove garlic, minced

☐ 1 teaspoon chopped fresh Italian parsley

☐ Dash black pepper

Directions

1. Trim broccoli, discarding tough stems. Cut broccoli into florets with 2-inch stems. Peel remaining stems; cut into ½-inch slices.

2. Bring 1 quart water to a boil in large saucepan over medium-high heat. Add broccoli; return to a boil. Cook 3 to 5 minutes or until broccoli is tender. Drain; transfer to serving dish.

3. Combine lemon juice, oil, garlic, parsley, and pepper in small bowl. Pour over broccoli; toss to coat. Cover and let stand 1 hour before serving to allow flavors to blend. Serve at room temperature.

Orange-Pomegranate Glazed Ham

Ingredients

☐ 1 (9 pound) bone-in, fully cooked, spiral-cut smoked ham half

☐ 1 cup pomegranate juice

☐ 3 tablespoons orange marmalade

☐ ¼ teaspoon ground cloves

☐ ½ teaspoon Dijon mustard

Directions

1. Preheat oven to 350°F. Unwrap ham; trim fat. Place, flat side down, on roasting pan. Cover loosely with foil. Bake 1 hour 45 minutes.

2. Meanwhile, heat juice in small saucepan over medium heat. Reduce heat to medium-low; cook 40 minutes or until juice is reduced to about 1/4 cup. Remove pan from heat. Let stand 10 minutes to cool slightly. Stir in marmalade, cloves, and mustard until smooth and well blended.

3. Remove foil from ham; brush evenly with orange-pomegranate glaze. Increase oven temperature to 425°F.

4. Bake 15 minutes. Let stand 5 minutes before slicing and serving.

Banana Blueberry Muffins – Nut Free

Ingredients

☐ 1 medium overripe banana mashed

☐ 3 eggs whisked

☐ 2 tbsp raw honey

☐ 1/3 cup full fat canned organic coconut milk

☐ 1 tsp pure vanilla extract

☐ ½ cup coconut flour

☐ 1 tbsp tapioca starch

☐ ½ tsp baking soda

☐ ½ tsp baking powder

☐ Pinch salt

☐ 2/3 cup fresh blueberries

Directions

1. Preheat your oven to 350 degrees and thoroughly grease a muffin pan with coconut oil or butter

2. In a medium bowl, combine the mashed banana, eggs, honey, coconut milk, and vanilla and beat until smooth

3. In a separate bowl, combine the coconut flour, tapioca, baking soda and powder, and salt.

4. Slowly stir the dry mix into the wet until fully combined. The coconut flour will make the batter thick.

5. Fold in the blueberries to combine. Fill your muffin cups about 2/3-3/4 full until all the batter is used up. I made 9 muffins with this recipe.

6. Bake in the preheated oven for 15-20 minutes or until lightly browned. Remove from oven, let sit for a minute and then remove muffins from pan to cool on a wire rack.

7. Perfect to eat warm or save for later. Enjoy!

9 798370 264511